Kettlebell
Home Workout for Beginners
+ Journal

Kettlebell Home Workout for Beginners plus Journal to track your kettlebell weight, reps, total volume, time, date, exercise, calories burned, heart rate, difficulty, how you felt, and other comments. All single kettlebell work and with warm-ups. Everything that you need to measure your progress and see results.

Everything is in simple language with great visuals that show exactly what needs to be done.

No fuzz, just the bare minimum of what you need to get started safely and make some serious progress. Simple but scalable so that even advanced users would get a real workout from this.

Workout name: **Beginners Workout by Cavemantraining**

Overall intensity: **Moderate**

Approx. total working time: **18 minutes**

Approx. total time with warm-up and rest: **30 minutes**

Overall benefits: **Strength, Cardio, Core**

Targets body parts: Arms, Back, Core, Glutes (Butt And Hips), Hamstrings (Back Of Upper Leg), Hips, Legs, Shoulders, Triceps (Back Of Upper Arms)

Kettlebell Home Workout for Beginners + Journal, 1st Edition

Published by Cavemantraining

www.cavemantraining.com

Copyright © 2022 by Cavemantraining

Cavemantraining also publishes its books in electronic formats. Some content that appears in print may not be available in electronic books or vice versa. If you bought this book in digital format, it is digitally signed and password protected with identifiable information.

TABLE OF CONTENTS

Programming (adjusting the workout to suit your needs)

The easy answer: Pick a weight that you can complete all rounds with and at nearly the same pace.

Your objective is to work at a steady pace for the full working time of each set and complete the last round with the same weight and number of reps for each set. Once you reach that point and are ready to progress, you can increase your weight if your goal is strength, or you can increase the working time from 45 to 60 seconds if your goal is endurance. You can also start adding rounds once it becomes really easy to complete the rounds.

How to pick the right kettlebell weight? You might only have one kettlebell available, work with that, but always make sure that you do not strain or injure yourself with a weight that is too heavy.

The complex answer: Once you are getting better at the workout and an exercise becomes easy, then you want to look at working in the right kettlebell weight range. To pick the right weight, you need to know your 1 repetition maximum (1RM) and work at the percentage around 40, 45, to 50% of your 1RM strict press.

Again, don't worry too much about this if you're just getting started. At first, your focus should be on form and technique, later you want to add speed, and then you want to look at strength. Once you're getting serious about strength, then you want to look at calculating your 1RM and working within that range. Over a long period, you want to look at increasing the weight as well.

If you can't maintain the right intensity/pace then you should adjust the weight and/or working time. If you only have one kettlebell then you would adjust the working time, i.e. from 45 to 30 seconds. If you have already adjusted the working time and still can't maintain a steady pace, then you are not working at the right pace, slow down your pace. A slower pace would mean that instead of performing 2 reps of a certain exercise in 5 seconds, you would only perform 1 rep in 5 seconds. This is just an example to show how to adjust the pace and doesn't necessarily reflect your pace.

Scoring (how to keep track of your progress)

Scoring is not recommended for beginners because the sole focus should be on form and technique. Once ready, your scoring is the total number of reps multiplied by your weight.

Scoring will become a big part of how you measure your progress, so, do keep it in the back of your mind. Of course, you can start keeping track of your scoring right away, however, it usually promotes going faster and heavier, which should not be your immediate focus as a beginner.

Scaling (how to adjust the workout)

The workout can be scaled by reducing the working time from 45 to 30 seconds and increasing the rest time from 15 to 30 seconds.

Reducing the working time from 45 to 30 seconds makes the workout easier. Increasing the resting time obviously provides you with more rest and thus makes the workout easier.

To make the workout harder, and as you progress you do want to make it harder, you increase the working time and potentially reduce or eventually remove the resting time.

Warm-up (preparing for the workout)

Raising the Temperature

Exercise(s) to perform:

3 × Bodyweight Hip Hinges (see further in this book)

3 × Squats (see further in this book but with no weight)

6 × Jumping Jacks

Perform the above sequence for 2 minutes and work at a moderate intensity and steady pace.

Perform joint work for 1 minute.

Create a circular pattern in the following joints: Wrists, shoulders, hips, ankles, and rotation in the thoracic spine rotations/circles. Start with a short range and increase the range as you get warmer and repeat the workout. Don't get too hung up on how to perform the joint work, as long as you are working on moving all those joints and trying to increase range, i.e. aiming to safely go further and become more flexible over time, then you are doing it right.

Perform 2 cycles of the whole warm-up, making a total of 6 minutes. If your environment is very cold, and you are very unconditioned, repeat the whole warm-up for 3 cycles (9 minutes).

Jumping Jack

A jumping jack is performed as following:

- Stand in a neutral position
- Arms hanging on the side
- Jump out to the side with the legs
- Raise the arms laterally overhead or into a V position
- The whole body looks like an X when viewing front on
- Return to the starting position

Workout Details

1st Exercise

The first exercise to perform is the Kettlebell Double Arm Swing for 45 seconds.

MAX reps (meaning to do as many as possible within the work time). Work at a moderate to vigorous intensity at a steady pace.

Rest for 15 seconds

2nd Exercise

The second exercise to perform is the Kettlebell Goblet Squat for 45 seconds. MAX reps and work at a moderate to vigorous intensity at a steady pace.

Rest for 15 seconds

3rd Exercise

The third exercise to perform is the Kettlebell Strict Press on one side for 45 seconds. MAX reps and work at a moderate to vigorous intensity at a steady pace.

Rest for 15 seconds

4th Exercise

The fourth exercise to perform is the Kettlebell Strict Press on the other side for 45 seconds. MAX reps and work at a moderate to vigorous intensity at a steady pace.

Rest for 15 seconds

5th Exercise

The fifth exercise to perform is the Kettlebell Split Stance Bent-Over Row on one side for 45 seconds. MAX reps and work at a moderate to vigorous intensity at a steady pace.

Rest for 15 seconds

6th Exercise

The sixth exercise to perform is the Kettlebell Split Stance Bent-Over Row on the other side for 45 seconds. MAX reps and work at a moderate to vigorous intensity at a steady pace.

Rest for 15 seconds

Rest

Active recovery for 1 minute consisting of stretching and/or mobility work. If you are just at the start of your journey, you might want to use the full minute for rest. As you get fitter, use this time to work on yourself with stretches. Don't get too hung up on how, as long as you are stretching the areas worked and working on improving range and mobility then you are doing it right.

The shoulders and triceps will be the areas that will need your attention the most.

Work at a light to moderate intensity and at a steady pace.

Note: This part can be skipped on the last round of the workout.

Complete 4 Rounds of the exercises which are 4.5 minutes work and 2.5 minutes rest each round, making a total of 18 minutes worked with 7.5 minutes rest.

If you are at the stage where you are scoring the workout, it's scored as Reps × Weight. You would record all your rep each round within the 15 seconds rest, add them all up at the end and multiply that by the weight used. This is your total scoring which you want to beat as you repeat the workout.

All exercises are explained further in the book.

Workout

45 seconds Kettlebell Double Arm Swing
15 seconds rest

45 seconds Kettlebell Goblet Squat
15 seconds rest

45 seconds Kettlebell Strict Press on one side
15 seconds rest

45 seconds Kettlebell Strict Press on the other side
15 seconds rest

45 seconds Kettlebell Split Stance Bent-Over Row on one side
15 seconds rest

Kettlebell Split Stance Bent-Over Row on the other side
15 seconds rest

1 minute of rest or active recovery

REPEAT 4 ROUNDS

Date: _____ **Kettlebell Weight:** _____

ROUND 1

Exercise:	1	2	3	4	5	6
Reps:						
Weight:						

ROUND 2

Exercise:	1	2	3	4	5	6
Reps:						
Weight:						

ROUND 3

Exercise:	1	2	3	4	5	6
Reps:						
Weight:						

ROUND 4

Exercise:	1	2	3	4	5	6
Reps:						
Weight:						

ROUND 5*

Exercise:	1	2	3	4	5	6
Reps:						
Weight:						

ROUND 6*

Exercise:	1	2	3	4	5	6
Reps:						
Weight:						

Completing this workout for the _____ time?

Work time _____ seconds   Rest time _____ seconds

Calories burned: _____   Difficulty: _____

Heart rate avg.: _____ BPM Heart rate high: _____   BPM

How do you feel?

_____

_____

_____

_____

How quickly did you recover during the 1-minute rest?

_____

_____

Total volume
Total Reps × Kettlebell Weight   _____

How did you feel the next day?

_____

_____

Comments:

_____

_____

_____

_____

_____

Date: _____   Kettlebell Weight: _____

ROUND 1

Exercise:	1	2	3	4	5	6
Reps:						
Weight:						

ROUND 2

Exercise:	1	2	3	4	5	6
Reps:						
Weight:						

ROUND 3

Exercise:	1	2	3	4	5	6
Reps:						
Weight:						

ROUND 4

Exercise:	1	2	3	4	5	6
Reps:						
Weight:						

ROUND 5*

Exercise:	1	2	3	4	5	6
Reps:						
Weight:						

ROUND 6*

Exercise:	1	2	3	4	5	6
Reps:						
Weight:						

Completing this workout for the _____ time?

Work time _____ seconds   Rest time _____ seconds

Calories burned: _____   Difficulty: _____

Heart rate avg.: _____   BPM Heart rate high: _____   BPM

How do you feel?

_____

_____

_____

_____

How quickly did you recover during the 1-minute rest?

_____

_____

Total volume
Total Reps × Kettlebell Weight   _____

How did you feel the next day?

_____

_____

Comments:

_____

_____

_____

_____

_____

Date: _____   Kettlebell Weight: _____

ROUND 1

Exercise:	1	2	3	4	5	6
Reps:						
Weight:						

ROUND 2

Exercise:	1	2	3	4	5	6
Reps:						
Weight:						

ROUND 3

Exercise:	1	2	3	4	5	6
Reps:						
Weight:						

ROUND 4

Exercise:	1	2	3	4	5	6
Reps:						
Weight:						

ROUND 5*

Exercise:	1	2	3	4	5	6
Reps:						
Weight:						

ROUND 6*

Exercise:	1	2	3	4	5	6
Reps:						
Weight:						

Completing this workout for the _____ time?

Work time _____ seconds   Rest time _____ seconds

Calories burned: _____   Difficulty: _____

Heart rate avg.: _____ BPM Heart rate high: _____ BPM

How do you feel?

_____

_____

_____

_____

How quickly did you recover during the 1-minute rest?

_____

_____

Total volume
Total Reps × Kettlebell Weight   _____

How did you feel the next day?

_____

_____

Comments:

_____

_____

_____

_____

_____

How to Keep Your Journal

If you used the same weight for the whole workout, you can record it only once at the top, but if you use different weights then you can record it for each exercise and round.

The work time is set to 45 seconds and the rest time to 15 seconds, but if you need to adjust that, the journal allows you to make note of that. At the start of your journey, start with 30 seconds to ease into it.

The difficulty allows you to make a short note of how difficult it felt to complete the workout. You can include more details about this under the notes. It's important to keep track of this as the difficulty will change and if you don't write it down you will not remember. When it becomes easier to complete the workout, you know that you're making progress. RPE stands for Rate of Perceived Exertion.

Rating	How the exertion feels
6	No exertion at all: doing nothing or resting
7.5	Extremely light exertion: slightly increased heart rate
9	Very light exertion: a gentle walk
11	Light exertion: a person has more than enough energy to continue exercising

13	Slightly hard exertion: exercising is getting more difficult but is still manageable
15	Hard exertion: continuing the activity is noticeably more difficult
17	Very hard exertion: a person can maintain this level of physical activity if they push themselves — they are very tired.
20	Maximal exertion: complete exhaustion

The heart rate entries are important to see how high your heart rate goes. How quickly does it go up? How long does it stay up? How quickly does it go down to a level of X BPM that feels like you're ok to go hard again? The quicker it goes down, the fitter you're getting. Again, an important factor to measure your progress. Are you still working at the same or a higher pace, with the same weight, getting more reps out, and your average heart rate is lower? You have made progress!

Are you feeling much better the next day or not feeling anything at all anymore? You've made progress.

*Note that the 5th and 6th round are included for when you progress and are ready to increase your rounds.

To reduce the cost of the book, I have only included three sheets of the journal for this workout, it didn't feel right to fill the book with many copies of the journal. You can scan or take a photo of the tables in which you'll log your entries and print duplicates, or you can download a file to print from our website here https://go.cavemantraining.com/printjournal

There is another version on Amazon that has more pages for the journal but is more expensive as they charge for more pages.

Kettlebell Exercises

Kettlebell Double Arm Swing

Key points:

- Use only the legs to move the weight
- Move the weight fast enough so the shoulders don't need to raise the weight
- Let the weight fall back down at the top and stand tall until it has passed approx. hip height
- Bend at the hips and knees while keeping the back straight and shoulders back
- Insert the weight between the legs
- Pull the weight out through the force of the legs
- Direct the weight in front
- Generate enough force with the legs to move the weight till approx. chest height
- Keep the shins vertical at all times
- Create a loose hook grip around the handle
- Do not grip the handle tightly
- Stand tall and tight at the top of the swing
- Compare your form and technique against the photos

Other objectives you can work towards outside of the workout with the swing are:

- Swinging heavier
- Swinging longer unbroken (pacing)

- Swinging higher volume (more total reps no matter whether the sets were broken)
- Swinging faster and with more explosive power (you need heavier weight for explosiveness)

Note: these other objectives take time to progress to, we're talking months, and within each objective you could be working for months. In other words, set your goals correctly, invest the time, and don't skip steps.

Kettlebell Swing

The shins should remain vertical at all times during a kettlebell swing that's performed with a hip hinge.

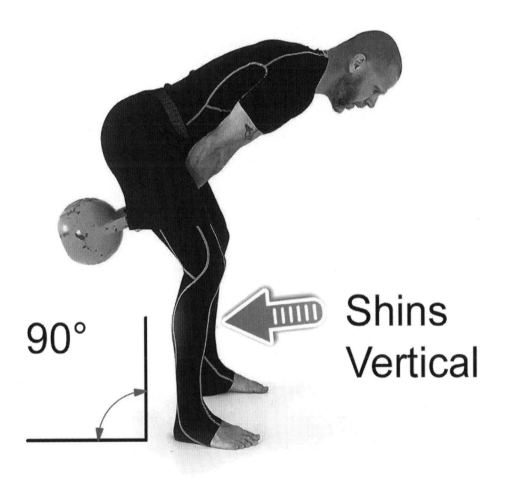

90°

Shins Vertical

The arms connect with the body as you insert the weight and the kettlebell remains an extension of the arms.

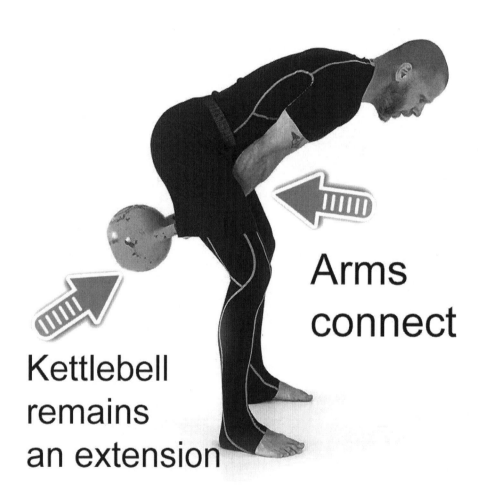

Arms
connect

Kettlebell
remains
an extension

The knees bend, and the hips are pushed back and down.

Hips are pushed back
and down

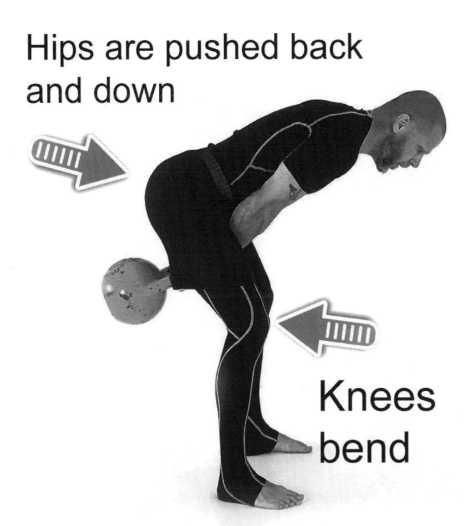

Knees
bend

The cervical (neck) remains in line with the rest of the spine.

The neck remains
in line with the
spine

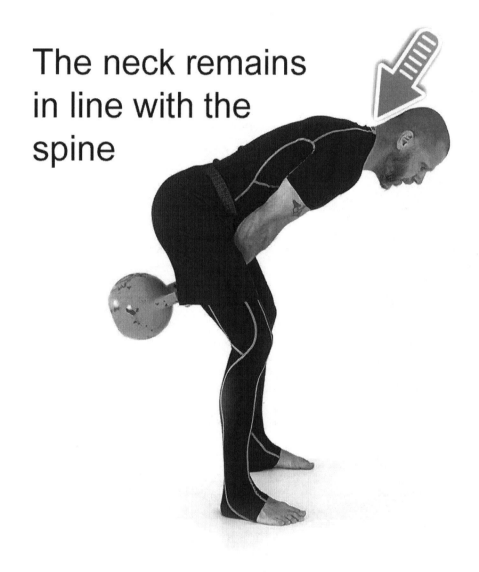

The elbows can be bent or straight. If bent, it has to be because of lat and chest activation, not because of actively pulling in with the elbow flexors (curling).

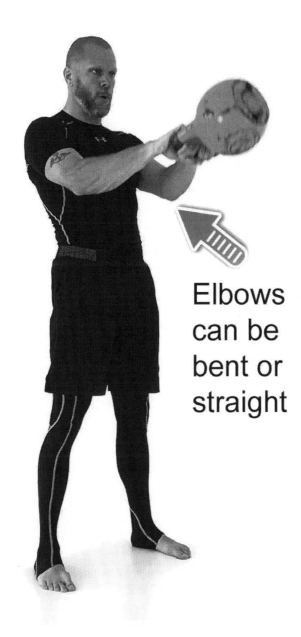

Elbows can be bent or straight

At the top of the swing, stand tall with the knees and hips straight (neutral position).

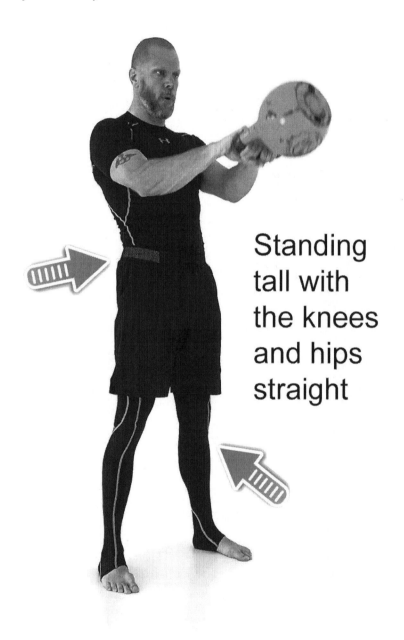

Standing
tall with
the knees
and hips
straight

Shoulders pulled down and away from the ears. The chest pushed out by pulling the scapula slightly together and down.

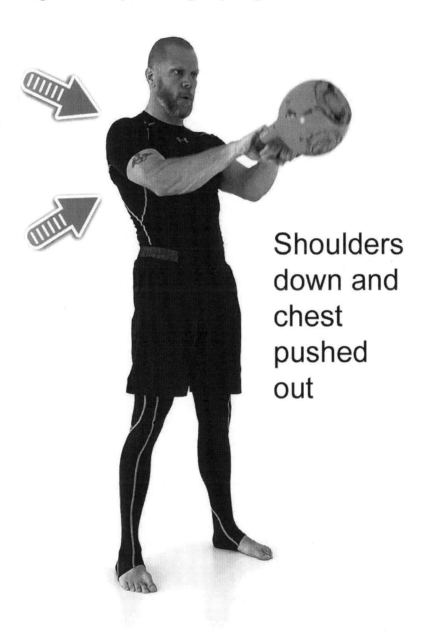

Shoulders down and chest pushed out

Hip Hinge

The hip hinge is the movement used for the kettlebell swing and also partly in the bent-over row.

The hip hinge is performed as:

- Stand in a neutral stance
- Keep the neck in line with the rest of the spine throughout the movement
- Keep the shins vertical throughout the movement
- The ankles are not moving
- The feet remain flat on the ground throughout the movement
- Let the arms hang loosely
- The spine stays straight throughout the movement
- Break and flex at the knees and hips
- Bringing the torso toward the ground but never past the hip line
- Push the hips slightly down and back during the movement
- It's normal to feel tension on the hamstrings as you move the hips back and down
- The bottom of the hip hinge:
- Eyesight is on the ground
- Shoulders are above the hip line and never lower than the hips
- The back is still straight
- The hips are pushed back and down
- The hips and knees are extended to stand back up
- The legs do the work and the torso just follows along

The next progression is to mimic the actual swing without weight as demonstrated in the following photos.

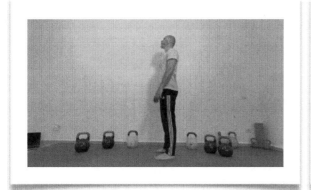
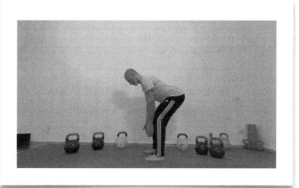
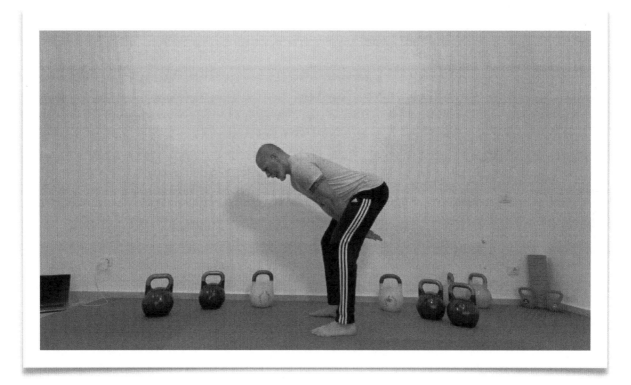

A) Stand in a neutral position.
B) Hinge at the hips and knees.
C) Insert the arms between the legs.

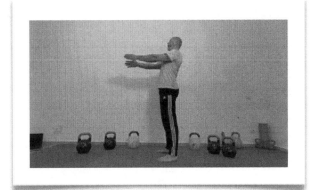 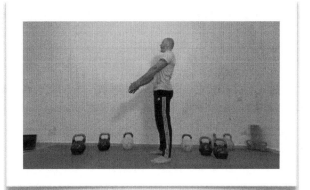

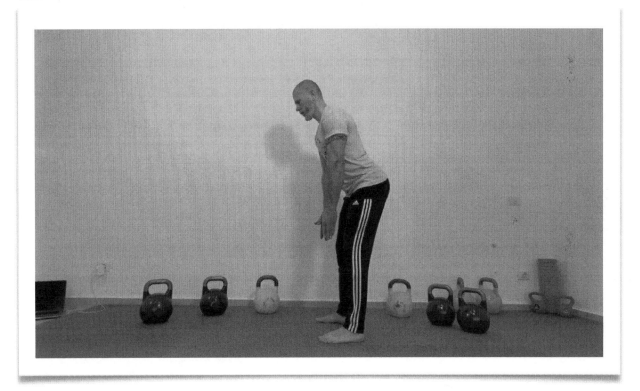

D) Stand straight with the arms out.

E) Remain in extension while the arms come down.
F) Hinge when the arms are near the legs.

Continue by inserting the arms through the legs so that the arms connect to the body.

The Swing is Lower-Body Powered

The swing is an all lower-body powered exercise. The following graphic shows what it would look like if the lower body is properly used to generate the force to move the weight.

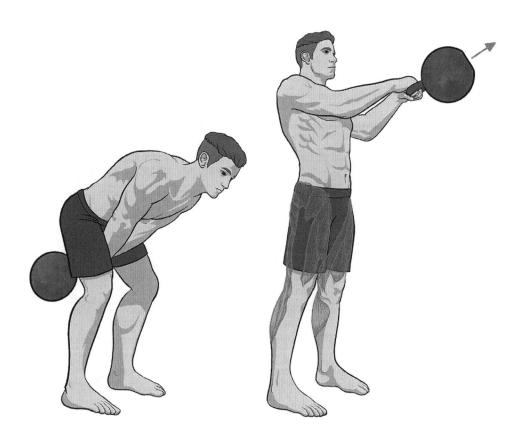

The following graphic shows what it would look like if the lower body is **not** used to generate the force to move the weight.

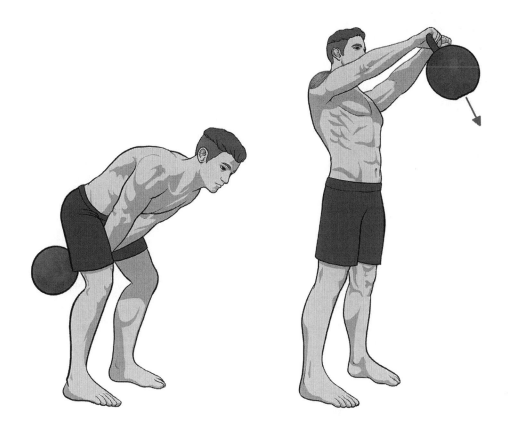

The kettlebell droops at the end of the swing when there is not enough force created by the legs and the arms start to raise the weight.

Kettlebell Goblet Squat

Key points:

- Break at three joints and let the hips lead going down
- Push yourself up starting at the feet
- Pull yourself up starting at the shoulders; i.e. let the shoulders lead going up
- Keep looking ahead
- Push the chest out and make sure the shoulder blades are doing their work
- Keep the elbows in nice and tight
- The knees can come over the toes as long as you keep the weight evenly distributed
- Maintain good form at all times
- Progress with depth/range over a period of time (go lower with better form as you repeat the workout)

Other objectives you can work towards outside of the workout with the squat are:

- Squat deeper (priority)
- Squat slower and more controlled (priority)
- Squat heavier (increasing strength)
- Squat longer unbroken (increasing muscular endurance)
- Squat higher volume
- Squat faster and with more explosive power (increasing speed and cardio)
- Squat double kettlebell

The elbows should be pulled in and positioned under the weight with the shoulders down.

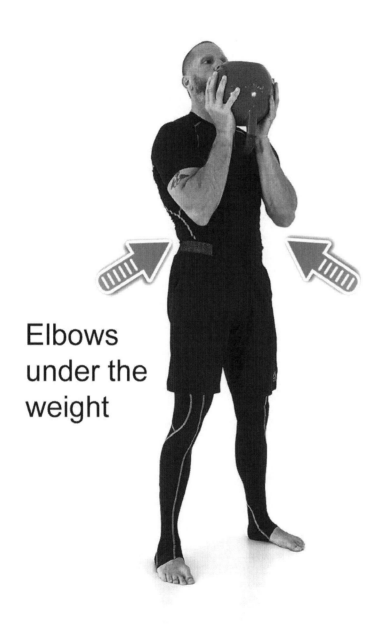

Elbows
under the
weight

The hips should come as low as possible and shoulders should stay high with the eye sight ahead.

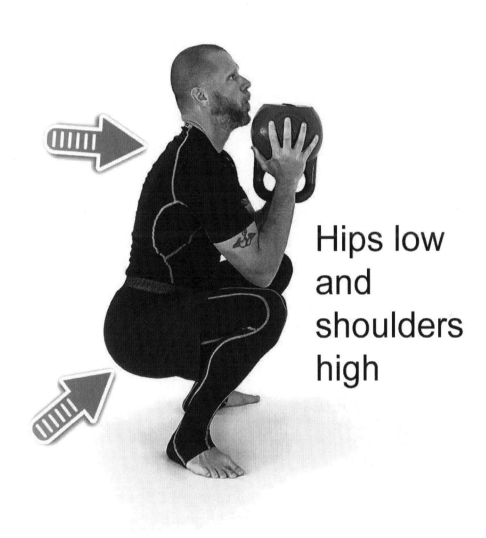

Hips low
and
shoulders

Keep the weight as close as is safely possible to the body.

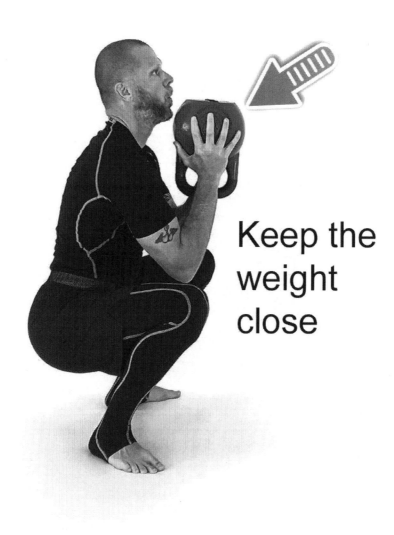

Keep the weight close

Kettlebell Strict Press

Key points:

- Keep everything firm while pressing
- Create a solid base to press from
- Use breathing and contraction of the muscles to create a solid structure to press from
- Only the elbow and shoulder should move
- Create tension on the non-pressing side by pulling the lat (latissimus dorsi) down and engaging the chest
- Keep the weight moving at the front for this stage of your journey

Other objectives you can work towards outside of the workout with the press are:

- Press slower and more controlled (priority)
- Press heavier
- Press longer unbroken
- Press higher volume
- Press double kettlebell

Keep the elbow positioned under the weight from start to finish.

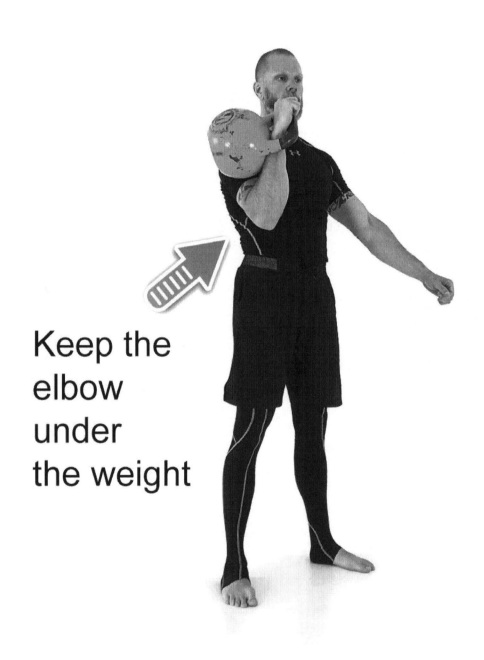

Keep the
elbow
under
the weight

Elbow straight (extended) and weight above the elbow and shoulder joint.

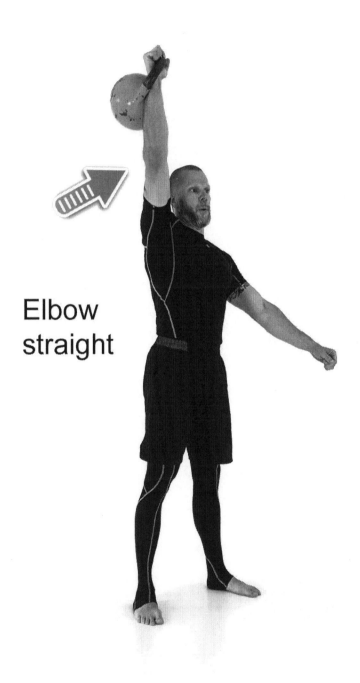

Elbow straight

Kettlebell Split Stance Bent-Over Row

Key points:

- Keep everything firm while rowing
- Create a solid base to row from
- Use breathing and contraction of the muscles to create a solid structure to row from
- Only the elbow and shoulder should move
- Let the lat and rear deltoid do the work
- Avoid curling the weight

Other objectives you can work towards outside of the workout with the row are:

- Row slower and more controlled (priority)
- Row heavier
- Row longer unbroken
- Row higher volume
- Row double kettlebell with a bent-over (hip hinge) stance

Focus on pulling the elbow back and up rather than the hand toward the shoulder.

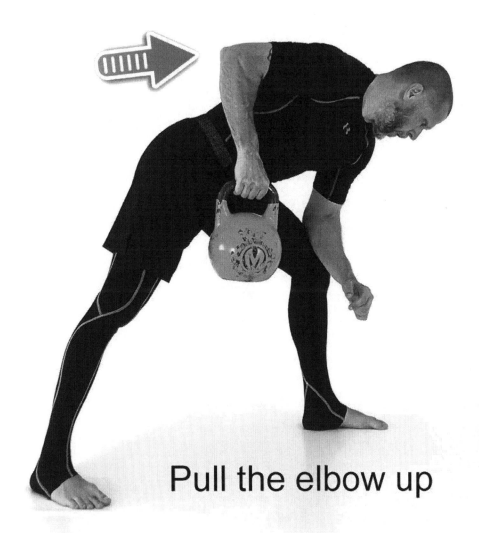

Pull the elbow up

Let the lower arm hang loosely and place the focus on the lat and rear deltoid to move the weight.

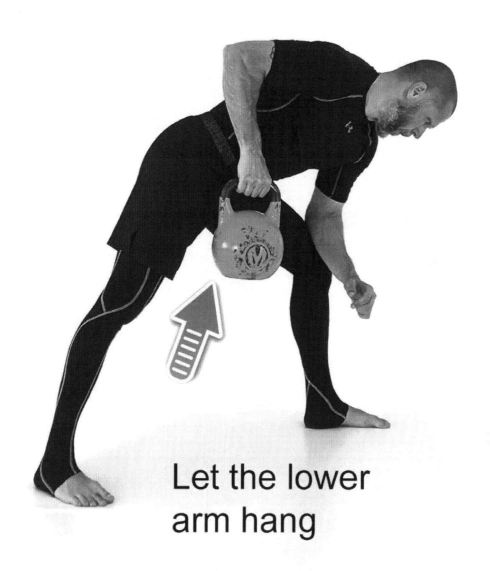

Let the lower
arm hang

Overall Tips

- Don't hold your breath
- Create tension on the inside to protect the spine when the load asks the most from your body
- Try to breathe out on every phase of an exercise
- Improve your form and technique before adding weight or anything else
- Improve your strength before adding speed
- Improve your range before adding volume or load

Use your breath to create tension on the inside. Try this, stand tall, and brace like someone is going to punch you in the stomach. Breathe in and push the air out through a little hole. Take note of how that feels inside, it feels different than just bracing your abdominals. Use this technique once you are ready to improve your breathing and training. Note, at the beginning of your journey you can't be focusing on too much at once as it becomes overbearing.

Shoulder mobility work

The following describes some of the movements to include for your mobility work. The harder the movement, the more you should include that in your programming. All work is to be performed slowly and controlled. Work on the sticking points. This means that when you're slowly moving from start to finish and you encounter a position that becomes awkward, difficult, or slightly painful, then you want to work and focus on that point until it's no longer awkward.

Shoulder circles

I use these regularly to loosen up my upper body and slowly add more movement top down. You can do them with both shoulders at once (in-sync), you can do them out of sync (offset), and one at a time to work on separation and mind-muscle connection.

A fancy term for shoulder circles is scapula elevation, scapula abduction, scapula depression, and scapula adduction. This movement involves a lot of muscles at the chest, neck, upper and lower back.

To perform:

- Stand in a neutral stance
- Pull the shoulders together at the front to separate the shoulder blades as much as possible
- Pull the shoulders down and away from the ears
- Activate the lats as well as the trapezius (lower); serratus anterior; and pectoralis minor
- Pull the shoulders back through scapulae adduction (pulling together)
- Pull the shoulders up toward the ears with the upper trapezius; rhomboids; and levator scapulae

Shoulder internal and external rotation

Internal and external shoulder rotation can also be referred to as shoulder medial rotation (internal) and shoulder lateral rotation (external). You can do this with the arms extended (straight) or with the arms flexed but for now, let's do them straight so we can focus on the direction of where the thumb points as that will make it easier to explain this exercise.

To perform:

- Stand in a neutral stance
- Arms hanging to the side
- Raise the arms laterally till just before shoulder height
- Palms facing down
- Your thumb is pointing forward
- Point the thumb to the back as far as possible
- Palms are now facing up
- Resist movement in the body
- Only the arm is rotating
- Perform the same movement in the other direction

Shoulder abduction

Abduction means to take away. We're taking away the arm from the midline of the body and we're also going to bring it into an overhead position. Not only is this just plain good for the shoulders but it's also going to help with your overhead work in kettlebell workouts, CrossFit, or any other training you do overhead. The key is to keep the body still, arms straight, and moving just a bit further every time. Once you have this movement under control you can start combining it with other exercises like the Hindu squat, reverse lunge, kneeling, etc. Combining this with other exercises usually digs deeper into the thoracic area, which is a good thing when you're ready for that.

To perform:

- Stand in a neutral stance
- Arms hanging beside you
- Elbows locked out through contraction of the triceps
- Press the heels into the ground to activate the hamstrings and pull down on the pelvis
- Squeeze the gluteus maximus to pull the pelvis from the top and keep it upright
- You can also contract the quads if you like for maximum body tension
- Brace your abs don't hold your breath
- Start abducting the shoulders
- Thumbs pointing laterally away from you (forearm supination) as you move up
- Engage the lats once you reach the shoulder line
- Pull the shoulder blades down
- Start pointing the thumbs back so that the palms can come flat together once max range has been reached
- Start pressing and pulling once overhead; press the hand to the sky and pull the arm down into its socket with the lats
- Think about pulling the biceps toward the ears
- Palms touching each other and press them together
- You're still pulling down while pressing up
- You can pair the overhead position with thoracic hyperextension

Your first goal is to get the hands above the shoulders, then thumbs touching each other, and from there you want to work on flat palms touching each other. All the tension throughout the body is required to create a stable base and most importantly protect the lumbar area from aches and pains. Thus, if you experience pains in the lower back you should look at whether you're contracting the right muscles to protect it by keeping the pelvis aligned with the spine, and secondly, you should look at whether your hip flexors are tight. Apart from safety, the tension is also great for just overall muscle control and creating strength through an isometric contraction. Why not benefit from the strength component when you're working on your shoulders right?

The ultimate goal of shoulder abduction to overhead is to get the palms touching each other with elbows locked out.

Shoulder flexion and extension

The meaning of flexion is easy to remember when you think about flexing the biceps. You're decreasing the angle in the elbow joint, decreasing the space between your hand and shoulder. With the knees, you're decreasing the angle in the knee joints, and decreasing the space between your heels and buttocks. With the hips, you're decreasing the angle in the hips, and decreasing the space between the shoulders and your feet. With the shoulders, it's a bit different as there is nothing on top to move towards. So, we're going to think about decreasing the angle between the elbow and head when looking side on, i.e. moving the upper arm toward being in line with the head.

Shoulder extension is the down part of when you've reached the max of shoulder flexion. Hyperextension is from the natural position of the arm, hanging, to the back. You won't get much range with hyperextension. To visualize extension think about standing in a neutral stance with the arms hanging beside you, not moving the body, and reaching for something behind you (rear delt contraction).

Performing this exercise is very similar to shoulder abduction when it comes to the tension/contraction you should maintain throughout the body while performing this move.

To perform:

- Arms hanging beside you
- Thumbs pointing forward/ahead
- Elbows locked out through contraction of the triceps
- Press the heels into the ground to activate the hamstrings and pull down on the pelvis
- Squeeze the gluteus maximus to pull the pelvis from the top and keep it upright
- You can also contract the quads for maximum body tension

- Brace your abs but don't hold your breath
- Start flexing one shoulder while hyperextending the other
- With the arm going overhead you also:
- Engage the lats once you reach the shoulder line
- Pull the shoulder blades down
- Once overhead start pressing and pulling; press the hand to the sky and pull the arm down into its socket with the lats
- Think about pulling the biceps toward the ear to keep the arm in line with the shoulder
- Alternate once you reach the extent for both arms

A simple way to describe this exercise is one arm up while the other is down and back. One shoulder is flexed while the other shoulder is extended.

Avoid Injury

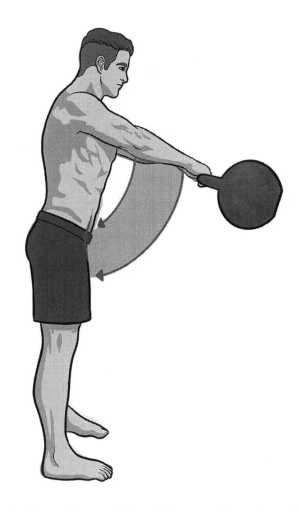

This graphic shows the early breaking at the hips on the drop for the backswing during kettlebell swings. Breaking early will bring the weight further away from the body and put unnecessary stress on the back. Remain straight until the weight is near the body as demonstrated in the following graphics.

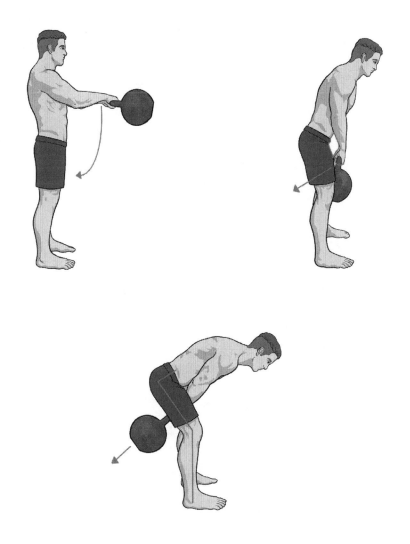

During the double-arm swing, you stay standing straight until the upper arms touch the body, whether that is the triceps touching your lats or some other part, that's the cue to starting hinging (see graphic 2). Hinge at the hips and direct the weight to the back (see graphic 3).

NB: The artist went a bit overboard with the development of the lats and upper back in the last position which makes it look like there is flexion in the upper back, there should not be any.

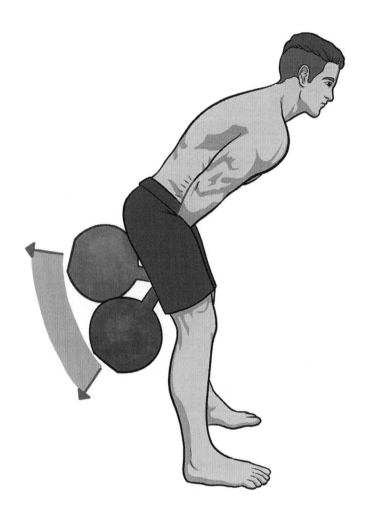

This is what I call bobbing of the kettlebell, a short abrupt movement at the end of the backswing because the body abruptly stops the arms but not the weight. This produces friction within the hands and can result in blisters or ripped hands over time. The solution to this is shown in the previous graphics.

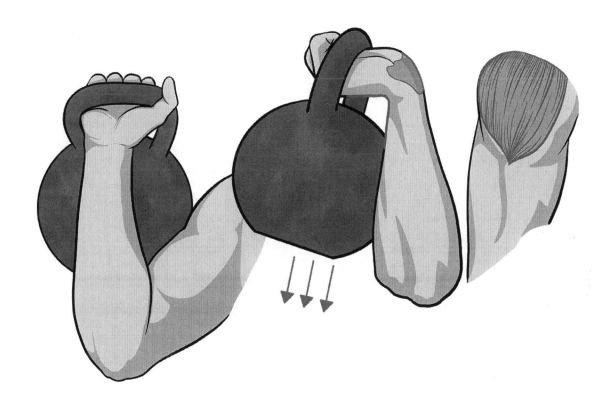

The graphic above shows an incorrect grip and racking position. The first graphic on the left shows how the handle is placed horizontally within the palm creating a broken wrist grip where the line is broken at the wrist. The broken wrist grip can be seen in the second graphic. The third graphic shows how this grip and racking mistake places additional stress on the deltoids.

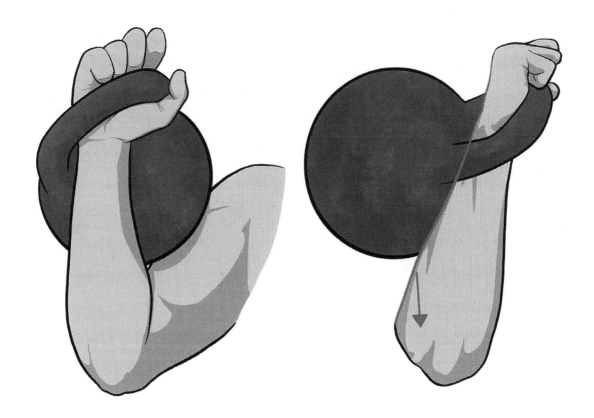

The graphic above shows the correct grip and racking position. A good 45-degree angle is achieved with hand insertion and the weight rest correctly on more than one point of contact.

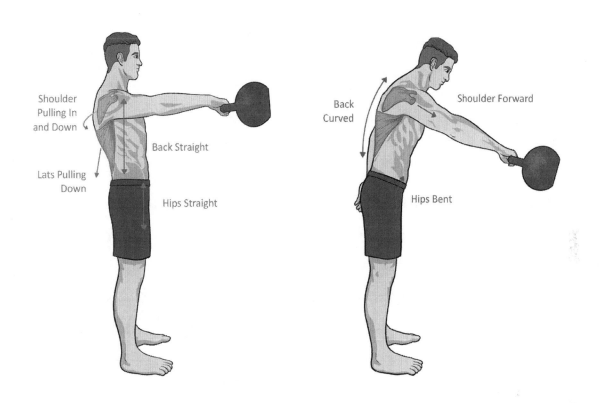

Shoulder Pulling In and Down

Back Straight

Lats Pulling Down

Hips Straight

Back Curved

Shoulder Forward

Hips Bent

The graphic above shows what the top of the swing should look like. The second graphic shows what following the kettlebell looks like, i.e. breaking too early at the hips.

Signs that indicate that what you're doing is too much or too heavy and/or that indicate that your technique needs to be improved:

- Lower back pains
- Grip/forearm aches and pains
- Excessive calluses
- Blisters

Lower back pain is never good, rest, recover, re-assess, modify, and start again.

Grip/forearm aches and pains are never good, rest, recover, re-assess, modify, and start again. Heed the warning signs in this area.

Calluses need to be maintained before they turn into cracked skin and open up.

Blisters occur through friction or sweat. Friction can be avoided by the correct technique.

What's Next?

After you have mastered the basic exercises for this kettlebell workout you're ready to explore more complex workouts with other kettlebell exercises. Do spend as much time on each new exercise that you did with this routine.

Look at kettlebell sport if you're after something that doesn't involve too many exercises but provides structure and competition. At Cavemantraining we have a whole course called Kettlebell Sport for Beginners and it breaks everything down even more than it did in this book.

If you want to work with something that will increase your mental toughness, strength, and endurance, look into THE PACE MAKER PROTOCOL. It's an awesome results-producing protocol.

If you want to focus on increasing your strength and muscle size, and have access to more than one kettlebell, look into Prometheus Phase II. It's a split workout that provides structure for 3, 4, or 6-days a week.

There are also the Kettlebell Workouts and Challenges 1, 2, and 3 books, perhaps even 4 by the time that you read this.

And last but not least, there is the Caveman Inner Circle, our online kettlebell workout library that comes with optional coaching from myself and other trainers. There are over 200 full-length follow-along workouts in there, including a follow-along session that breaks down the technique for the workout in this book, covers common mistakes, alternatives and progressions, and the click-and-play videos for the warm-up and cooldown. Also available with a premium membership to the Kettlebell Exercise Encyclopedia.

You can find all the above-mentioned products at www.cavemantraining.com/shop or just email info@cavemantraining.com and someone will reply within 24 hours.

You can join our online communities for free and post your results, discuss any issues, boost about your progress, ask for feedback, or discuss kettlebells in general. You can join our communities here go.cavemantraining.com/social

You can also record your scoring publicly on our Kettlebell Exercise Encyclopedia, which makes it easy to have all your scoring in one handy place. https://kettlebellexercises.fitness

About the Author

My name is Taco Fleur. The first thing I'd like you to know about me is that I do not know everything, I don't pretend to know everything, and I never will. I'm on a path of lifelong learning. I believe there is always something to learn from someone, no matter who they are.

I've been physically active since the day I arrived on this earth in 1973. I got serious about training in 1999, touched a kettlebell for the first time in 2004, and got serious about kettlebell training in 2009. I'm here to do what I love most, and that is to share my knowledge with the world.

Some of my qualifications are:

- Russian Girevoy Sport Institute Kettlebell Coach
- IKFF Certified Kettlebell Teacher
- Kettlebell Sport Rank 2
- HardstyleFit Kettlebell Level 1 Instructor
- CrossFit Level 1 Trainer
- CrossFit Judges Certificate
- CrossFit Lesson Planning Certificate
- Kettlebells Level 2 Trainer
- Kettlebell Science and Application
- MMA Fitness Level 2
- MMA Conditioning Level 1
- BJJ Purple Belt
- and more...

Owner of Cavemantraining, Kettlebell University, and Kettlebell Training Education. Author on BoxRox. Featured in 4 issues of the Iron Man magazine. I have owned and set up 3 functional kettlebell gyms in Australia and Vietnam, and lived in the Netherlands, Australia, Vietnam, Thailand, Italy, Tanzania, Albania, and I'm currently living in Greece.

Some of my **personal bests** are:

- 1 hour unbroken clean and jerk with a 16kg
- 45 minutes unbroken clean and jerk with a 20kg
- 400 burpees performed within one hour
- 500 kettlebell snatches, 500 swings, and 500 double-unders completed in one session
- 250 alternating dead clean and presses in one session with 20kg
- 200 pull-ups in one session
- 200 unbroken kettlebell swings with a 28kg
- Most kettlebell swings completed in one session with a 28kg (1,501)
- Most total kettlebell swings completed in 28 days with a 28kg (11,111)
- Windmill with a 40kg kettlebell
- Chest press with two 40kg dumbbells (total 80kg)
- Lugged a 16kg kettlebell up a 3,479m mountain
- 160kg deadlift
- 50 CrossFit Burpees and 100 single-arm swings unbroken in 5:34
- 100 snatches on sand with a 24kg kettlebell
- 85kg Olympic Squat Snatch
- 300 unbroken clean and jerk with 20kg kettlebell
- 10 minute unbroken clean and jerk 80 reps with 2 × 16kg kettlebells
- 532 unbroken snatches and achieved rank 2 in kettlebell sport

I mention these PBs not to boast but to demonstrate that I have a good understanding of technique and movement across different areas.

My own training and goals are geared around GPP (General Physical Preparedness), which involves kettlebell training, calisthenics, mobility, and

CrossFit. I like high-volume reps but also like greasing the groove now and again. My main goals are to remain as agile and mobile as possible, to train in as many planes of movement as possible, and to learn as many different exercise combinations and movements as possible while having fun and enjoying other ways of movement such as Brazilian Jiu-Jitsu. I'm no Arnold Schwarzenegger and never will be, but strength is not solely defined by physical appearance and huge bulging muscles.

You can read more about my training, philosophy, and other ramblings on the Cavemantraining website, www.cavemantraining.com, and on the Cavemantraining YouTube channel, www.youtube.com/Cavemantraining, which as of this writing has over 61,600 subscribers and more than 20 million views.

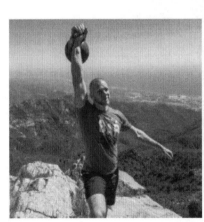 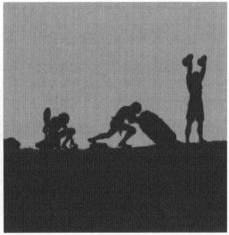 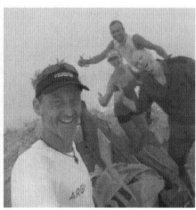

Facebook.com/**coach.taco.fleur** for detailed moves and tips
Facebook.com/**Cavemantraining** for up-to-date articles and news
Instagram: *@realcavemantraining*
Reddit: *u/cavemankettlebells*

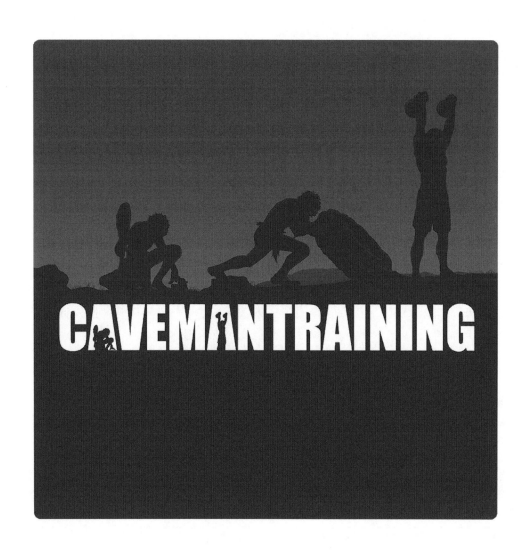

Other Books

Other books or products by Cavemantraining that you will enjoy are:

- Private coaching and 180+ online kettlebell library for less than the cost of two cups of coffee at Starbucks per week.
  go.cavemantraining.com/cic
- Buy kettlebell workout videos
  www.cavemantraining.com/buy-kettlebell-workouts/
- Become kettlebell certified online
  www.cavemantraining.com/online-kettlebell-courses-and-certifications/
- Buy kettlebell workout books
  www.cavemantraining.com/product-category/kettlebell-books/
- 3 or 4-Day Kettlebell Split Strength Program
  www.cavemantraining.com/shop/kettlebells/kettlebell-4-day-split-strength-program/
- And so much more
  www.cavemantraining.com/shop/

THANKS

A special thanks to:

- everyone that's reading, wanting to learn about kettlebells, and looking for the best kettlebell workouts as you give me purpose.
- everyone who has trained with me in person, seeing your progression is what gives me joy.
- everyone participating in our kettlebell communities, it's you who's asking questions that prompts me to explore more and to make sure that I keep verifying that the education I spread is the right one.
- the kettlebell, you give me the enthusiasm to keep exploring, not only with technique and exercises, but most of all when dragging kettlebells to places no kettlebell has gone before.
- my wife, son, and dog for accompanying me on many adventures and workouts across the world.

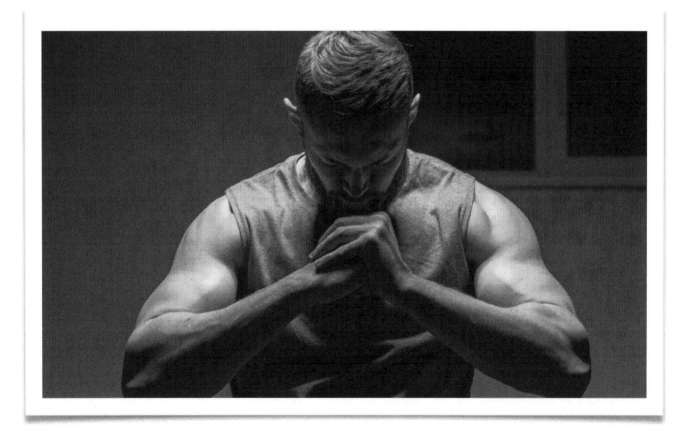

Kettlebell Communities

Cavemantraining runs many online kettlebell communities and I would love to see you post in any of them about your results with the Beginners Workout by Cavemantraining.

Come and join us here go.cavemantraining.com/social

Make sure to subscribe to our YouTube channel as well youtube.com/cavemantraining

THE END

Date: _____   Kettlebell Weight: _____

ROUND 1

Exercise:	1	2	3	4	5	6
Reps:						
Weight:						

ROUND 2

Exercise:	1	2	3	4	5	6
Reps:						
Weight:						

ROUND 3

Exercise:	1	2	3	4	5	6
Reps:						
Weight:						

ROUND 4

Exercise:	1	2	3	4	5	6
Reps:						
Weight:						

ROUND 5*

Exercise:	1	2	3	4	5	6
Reps:						
Weight:						

ROUND 6*

Exercise:	1	2	3	4	5	6
Reps:						
Weight:						

Completing this workout for the _____ time?

Work time _____ seconds   Rest time _____ seconds

Calories burned: _____   Difficulty: _____

Heart rate avg.: _____ BPM Heart rate high: _____ BPM

How do you feel?

_____

_____

_____

_____

How quickly did you recover during the 1-minute rest?

_____

_____

Total volume
Total Reps × Kettlebell Weight   _____

How did you feel the next day?

_____

_____

Comments:

_____

_____

_____

_____

_____

Date: _____ Kettlebell Weight: _____

ROUND 1

Exercise:	1	2	3	4	5	6
Reps:						
Weight:						

ROUND 2

Exercise:	1	2	3	4	5	6
Reps:						
Weight:						

ROUND 3

Exercise:	1	2	3	4	5	6
Reps:						
Weight:						

ROUND 4

Exercise:	1	2	3	4	5	6
Reps:						
Weight:						

ROUND 5*

Exercise:	1	2	3	4	5	6
Reps:						
Weight:						

ROUND 6*

Exercise:	1	2	3	4	5	6
Reps:						
Weight:						

Completing this workout for the _____ time?

Work time _____ seconds   Rest time _____ seconds

Calories burned: _____   Difficulty: _____

Heart rate avg.: _____ BPM Heart rate high: _____ BPM

How do you feel?

_____

_____

_____

_____

How quickly did you recover during the 1-minute rest?

_____

_____

Total volume
Total Reps × Kettlebell Weight   _____

How did you feel the next day?

_____

_____

Comments:

_____

_____

_____

_____

_____

Date: _____   Kettlebell Weight: _____

ROUND 1

Exercise:	1	2	3	4	5	6
Reps:						
Weight:						

ROUND 2

Exercise:	1	2	3	4	5	6
Reps:						
Weight:						

ROUND 3

Exercise:	1	2	3	4	5	6
Reps:						
Weight:						

ROUND 4

Exercise:	1	2	3	4	5	6
Reps:						
Weight:						

ROUND 5*

Exercise:	1	2	3	4	5	6
Reps:						
Weight:						

ROUND 6*

Exercise:	1	2	3	4	5	6
Reps:						
Weight:						

Completing this workout for the _____ time?

Work time _____ seconds   Rest time _____ seconds

Calories burned: _____   Difficulty: _____

Heart rate avg.: _____ BPM Heart rate high: _____ BPM

How do you feel?

_____

_____

_____

_____

How quickly did you recover during the 1-minute rest?

_____

_____

Total volume
Total Reps × Kettlebell Weight   _____

How did you feel the next day?

_____

_____

Comments:

_____

_____

_____

_____

_____

Date: _____   Kettlebell Weight: _____

ROUND 1

Exercise:	1	2	3	4	5	6
Reps:						
Weight:						

ROUND 2

Exercise:	1	2	3	4	5	6
Reps:						
Weight:						

ROUND 3

Exercise:	1	2	3	4	5	6
Reps:						
Weight:						

ROUND 4

Exercise:	1	2	3	4	5	6
Reps:						
Weight:						

ROUND 5*

Exercise:	1	2	3	4	5	6
Reps:						
Weight:						

ROUND 6*

Exercise:	1	2	3	4	5	6
Reps:						
Weight:						

Completing this workout for the _____ time?

Work time _____ seconds   Rest time _____ seconds

Calories burned: _____   Difficulty: _____

Heart rate avg.: _____ BPM Heart rate high: _____ BPM

How do you feel?

_____

_____

_____

_____

How quickly did you recover during the 1-minute rest?

_____

_____

Total volume
Total Reps × Kettlebell Weight   _____

How did you feel the next day?

_____

_____

Comments:

_____

_____

_____

_____

_____

Date: _____   Kettlebell Weight: _____

ROUND 1

Exercise:	1	2	3	4	5	6
Reps:						
Weight:						

ROUND 2

Exercise:	1	2	3	4	5	6
Reps:						
Weight:						

ROUND 3

Exercise:	1	2	3	4	5	6
Reps:						
Weight:						

ROUND 4

Exercise:	1	2	3	4	5	6
Reps:						
Weight:						

ROUND 5*

Exercise:	1	2	3	4	5	6
Reps:						
Weight:						

ROUND 6*

Exercise:	1	2	3	4	5	6
Reps:						
Weight:						

Completing this workout for the _____ time?

Work time _____ seconds   Rest time _____ seconds

Calories burned: _____   Difficulty: _____

Heart rate avg.: _____ BPM Heart rate high: _____ BPM

How do you feel?

_____

_____

_____

_____

How quickly did you recover during the 1-minute rest?

_____

_____

Total volume
Total Reps × Kettlebell Weight   _____

How did you feel the next day?

_____

_____

Comments:

_____

_____

_____

_____

_____

Date: _____   **Kettlebell Weight:** _____

ROUND 1

Exercise:	1	2	3	4	5	6
Reps:						
Weight:						

ROUND 2

Exercise:	1	2	3	4	5	6
Reps:						
Weight:						

ROUND 3

Exercise:	1	2	3	4	5	6
Reps:						
Weight:						

ROUND 4

Exercise:	1	2	3	4	5	6
Reps:						
Weight:						

      Copyright Cavemantraining 2022

ROUND 5*

Exercise:	1	2	3	4	5	6
Reps:						
Weight:						

ROUND 6*

Exercise:	1	2	3	4	5	6
Reps:						
Weight:						

Completing this workout for the _____ time?

Work time _____ seconds   Rest time _____ seconds

Calories burned: _____   Difficulty: _____

Heart rate avg.: _____ BPM Heart rate high: _____ BPM

How do you feel?

_____

_____

_____

_____

How quickly did you recover during the 1-minute rest?

_____

_____

Total volume
Total Reps × Kettlebell Weight   _____

How did you feel the next day?

_____

_____

Comments:

_____

_____

_____

_____

_____

Date: _____   Kettlebell Weight: _____

ROUND 1

Exercise:	1	2	3	4	5	6
Reps:						
Weight:						

ROUND 2

Exercise:	1	2	3	4	5	6
Reps:						
Weight:						

ROUND 3

Exercise:	1	2	3	4	5	6
Reps:						
Weight:						

ROUND 4

Exercise:	1	2	3	4	5	6
Reps:						
Weight:						

ROUND 5*

Exercise:	1	2	3	4	5	6
Reps:						
Weight:						

ROUND 6*

Exercise:	1	2	3	4	5	6
Reps:						
Weight:						

Completing this workout for the _____ time?

Work time _____ seconds   Rest time _____ seconds

Calories burned: _____   Difficulty: _____

Heart rate avg.: _____ BPM Heart rate high: _____ BPM

How do you feel?

_____

_____

_____

_____

How quickly did you recover during the 1-minute rest?

_____

_____

Total volume
Total Reps × Kettlebell Weight   _____

How did you feel the next day?

_____

_____

Comments:

_____

_____

_____

_____

_____

Date: _____   Kettlebell Weight: _____

ROUND 1

Exercise:	1	2	3	4	5	6
Reps:						
Weight:						

ROUND 2

Exercise:	1	2	3	4	5	6
Reps:						
Weight:						

ROUND 3

Exercise:	1	2	3	4	5	6
Reps:						
Weight:						

ROUND 4

Exercise:	1	2	3	4	5	6
Reps:						
Weight:						

ROUND 5*

Exercise:	1	2	3	4	5	6
Reps:						
Weight:						

ROUND 6*

Exercise:	1	2	3	4	5	6
Reps:						
Weight:						

Completing this workout for the _____ time?

Work time _____ seconds   Rest time _____ seconds

Calories burned: _____   Difficulty: _____

Heart rate avg.: _____ BPM Heart rate high: _____ BPM

How do you feel?

_____

_____

_____

_____

How quickly did you recover during the 1-minute rest?

_____

_____

Total volume
Total Reps × Kettlebell Weight   _____

How did you feel the next day?

_____

_____

Comments:

_____

_____

_____

_____

_____

Date: _____ Kettlebell Weight: _____

ROUND 1

Exercise:	1	2	3	4	5	6
Reps:						
Weight:						

ROUND 2

Exercise:	1	2	3	4	5	6
Reps:						
Weight:						

ROUND 3

Exercise:	1	2	3	4	5	6
Reps:						
Weight:						

ROUND 4

Exercise:	1	2	3	4	5	6
Reps:						
Weight:						

ROUND 5*

Exercise:	1	2	3	4	5	6
Reps:						
Weight:						

ROUND 6*

Exercise:	1	2	3	4	5	6
Reps:						
Weight:						

Completing this workout for the _____ time?

Work time _____ seconds   Rest time _____ seconds

Calories burned: _____   Difficulty: _____

Heart rate avg.: _____ BPM Heart rate high: _____ BPM

How do you feel?

_____

_____

_____

_____

How quickly did you recover during the 1-minute rest?

_____

_____

Total volume
Total Reps × Kettlebell Weight   _____

How did you feel the next day?

_____

_____

Comments:

_____

_____

_____

_____

_____

Date: _____   Kettlebell Weight: _____

ROUND 1

Exercise:	1	2	3	4	5	6
Reps:						
Weight:						

ROUND 2

Exercise:	1	2	3	4	5	6
Reps:						
Weight:						

ROUND 3

Exercise:	1	2	3	4	5	6
Reps:						
Weight:						

ROUND 4

Exercise:	1	2	3	4	5	6
Reps:						
Weight:						

ROUND 5*

Exercise:	1	2	3	4	5	6
Reps:						
Weight:						

ROUND 6*

Exercise:	1	2	3	4	5	6
Reps:						
Weight:						

Completing this workout for the _____ time?

Work time _____ seconds   Rest time _____ seconds

Calories burned: _____   Difficulty: _____

Heart rate avg.: _____ BPM Heart rate high: _____ BPM

How do you feel?

_____

_____

_____

_____

How quickly did you recover during the 1-minute rest?

_____

_____

Total volume
Total Reps × Kettlebell Weight   _____

How did you feel the next day?

_____

_____

Comments:

_____

_____

_____

_____

_____

Date: _____   Kettlebell Weight: _____

ROUND 1

Exercise:	1	2	3	4	5	6
Reps:						
Weight:						

ROUND 2

Exercise:	1	2	3	4	5	6
Reps:						
Weight:						

ROUND 3

Exercise:	1	2	3	4	5	6
Reps:						
Weight:						

ROUND 4

Exercise:	1	2	3	4	5	6
Reps:						
Weight:						

ROUND 5*

Exercise:	1	2	3	4	5	6
Reps:						
Weight:						

ROUND 6*

Exercise:	1	2	3	4	5	6
Reps:						
Weight:						

Completing this workout for the _____ time?

Work time _____ seconds   Rest time _____ seconds

Calories burned: _____   Difficulty: _____

Heart rate avg.: _____ BPM Heart rate high: _____ BPM

How do you feel?

_____

_____

_____

_____

How quickly did you recover during the 1-minute rest?

_____

_____

Total volume
Total Reps × Kettlebell Weight _____

How did you feel the next day?

_____

_____

Comments:

_____

_____

_____

_____

_____

Date: _____   Kettlebell Weight: _____

ROUND 1

Exercise:	1	2	3	4	5	6
Reps:						
Weight:						

ROUND 2

Exercise:	1	2	3	4	5	6
Reps:						
Weight:						

ROUND 3

Exercise:	1	2	3	4	5	6
Reps:						
Weight:						

ROUND 4

Exercise:	1	2	3	4	5	6
Reps:						
Weight:						

ROUND 5*

Exercise:	1	2	3	4	5	6
Reps:						
Weight:						

ROUND 6*

Exercise:	1	2	3	4	5	6
Reps:						
Weight:						

Completing this workout for the _____ time?

Work time _____ seconds   Rest time _____ seconds

Calories burned: _____   Difficulty: _____

Heart rate avg.: _____ BPM Heart rate high: _____ BPM

How do you feel?

_____

_____

_____

_____

How quickly did you recover during the 1-minute rest?

_____

_____

Total volume
Total Reps × Kettlebell Weight _____

How did you feel the next day?

_____

_____

Comments:

_____

_____

_____

_____

_____

Made in the USA
Columbia, SC
12 August 2024

ed452e65-5589-4e0b-b6d0-c879e609b80eR01